UNDERSTANDING YOUR BLOODWORK AND HOW IT RELATES TO YOUR HEALTH ISSUES!

A REFERENCE GUIDE FOR PATIENTS

DR. STRONG D.C. DACNB,CFMP, PAK

CONTENTS

Introduction 7

About the Author 11

A Few Tips for Before, During, and After 13
Drawing Blood for Your Tests

The Complete Blood Count Panel - CBC 15

Iron Tests 30

The Basic Metabolic Panel - BMP 36

The Lipid (Fats) Panel 53

The Liver Panel 60

The Thyroid Panel 71

Testing for Inflammatory Markers 77

LIMITS OF LIABILITY/DISCLAIMER OF WARRANTY

Move towards optimal health now...

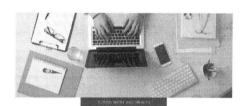

What's included?

- A complete 2-week sample diet
- Easy, tasty, health meals
- Optimize your bloodwork and health NOW!

To receive your 2-week sample diet, visit

https://bit.ly/2YmxBtn

INTRODUCTION

The goal of functional medicine is to examine a person and their body as a holistic system in order to discover and treat the root cause of any chronic conditions that are present. Once the root cause(s) is discovered, then the symptoms – **headaches, fatigue, depression, autoimmune disease** – may be treated effectively.

To get an accurate picture of your health, we have to start by running a series of "diagnostics" to see where you stand. Obtain a baseline, if you will. The best way to do this is with one or more blood tests designed to measure a variety of diagnostic points in different systems of your body – your immune system, adrenal system, and circulatory system, for example.

Once we have these results, we're able to review them and create a plan that will allow us to move forward on the right path of treatment. One of my goals as a functional medicine practitioner is to **empower you to take control of your health**.

I believe that if we focus on your health, your health issues go away. The goal of this guide in particular is to be a **comprehensive, yet simple way to help you understand what your clinical blood test results mean** and how you can work with your healthcare provider(s) to use this information to improve your health.

While this is not a substitute for the advice of a medical practitioner, you may use this as an initial tool and reference guide for reviewing test results. It may also serve as a resource that allows you to communicate more effectively with your healthcare providers about your overall health. You may also find that functional medicine standards interpret some ranges differently than "traditional" health care providers.

Inside, we'll cover the following tests/panels:

- Complete Blood Count Panel
- Basic Metabolic Panel
- Lipid Panel
- Liver Panel
- Thyroid Panel
- Iron Testing
- Inflammatory Marker Testing

- Urinalysis

In each section, you'll learn:

- What each test is used for
- Simple definitions on each diagnostic measurement point
- Clinical, optimal, and at-risk ranges for each point
- Note: a clinical range describes the normal standard for what the traditional healthcare model deems a regular range. This range is different from a functional medicine range, in that it does not necessarily proactively identify the development of potential disease.
- Common causes of irregular range measurements
- Supplement recommendations to support your body

A couple of things to remember:

- Your body is complex, and even if you see something that could be concerning on your test, make sure you consult your doctor and don't self-diagnose.
- This guide does not replace the expertise of a doctor. Again, please don't use this to self-diagnose, but as a starting point to understand your levels, and as a reference guide when your doctor is not available.

That being said, I hope this is an effective and valuable tool for you, and that it gives you confidence in understanding what your test results mean and how you can use them to improve and optimize your health.

ABOUT THE AUTHOR

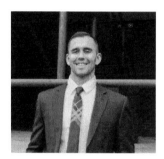

Dr. Todd Strong is a certified functional medicine practitioner based in Tennessee. His comprehensive training as an applied kinesiologist, board-certified chiropractor, and chiropractic neurologist provide a unique treatment perspective and methodology that truly helps patients heal and achieve optimal health.

Dr. Strong's specialty is working with patients to discover and treat underlying causes of chronic conditions such as fibromyalgia, chronic fatigue syndrome, headaches, multiple sclerosis, diabetes, hypertension, depression and anxiety, acid reflux, and others.

He believes that in empowering individuals to take control of their health and wellness, and his approach to treatment includes patient education – one of the most powerful tools medical practitioners have to help people resolve their health issues.

For more information and access to additional resources, please visit:

https://www.stronghealthinstitute.com

A FEW TIPS FOR BEFORE, DURING, AND AFTER DRAWING BLOOD FOR YOUR TESTS

1. For **cholesterol** and **glucose** tests, you must fast for at least 8 hours prior to having your blood drawn, unless your doctor tells you otherwise. Fasting means no eating or drinking for at least 8 hours before the test, except water. After your blood is drawn, you may resume your regular diet.

2. Drink plenty of water before your **blood test**. This helps keep your blood pressure from dropping. The leading cause of fainting and dizziness during a blood test is a drop in blood pressure. Avoid coffee or other caffeinated drinks before your test because they actually cause your body to expel water.

3. Unless fasting is required for your testing, eat breakfast to help keep your blood sugar up. This will help you feel better after your blood draw and prevent lightheadedness and dizziness. If you think you might

be nauseous during the blood draw, don't eat immediately before your appointment.

4. If you take a blood-thinning medication, such as heparin or Coumadin (warfarin), tell the phlebotomist about these medications before your blood is drawn. After your blood is drawn, the phlebotomist will closely observe the puncture site to see that bleeding has stopped before you leave the collection location.

5. Relax. If you are anxious about what is going to take place, ask the person taking your blood to explain everything he or she is doing. Or think of something entirely different, like your vacation or what you are going to do after your blood test. Ask a friend or loved one to go along with you if you feel that will help.

6. Eat a snack after you have your blood drawn. Take a snack with you if you will not be going directly back home or to work. That way you can eat it directly after the blood draw.

7. Your bandage can be removed after an hour. An easy way to remove the bandage is to loosen it after a bath or shower. If the area does bleed later, apply slight pressure until the bleeding stops and apply a new bandage. Bruising may occur at the blood draw site.Don't worry if this happens - apply some ice to the site and give it a few days to get better.

THE COMPLETE BLOOD COUNT
PANEL - CBC

A CBC (Complete Blood Count) Panel, also known as an FBC (full blood count) Panel is a standard lab test that gives important information about the cells in your blood. It's often ordered for healthy people as part of a medical examination and can also be used to help monitor or diagnose various health conditions.

Conditions such as anemia and thrombocytopenia can be diagnosed from abnormal results on the complete blood count. Certain results can indicate a need for urgent medical treatment, such as a blood transfusion if the hemoglobin is very low. Other results can help guide healthcare providers towards a diagnosis: for example, the red blood cell indices can provide information about the cause of a person's anemia. Complete blood count results are interpreted by comparing them to reference ranges, which vary based on sex and age.

The test reports on: amounts of: white blood cell count and differential (counts the different types of white blood cells), red blood cell count, concentration of hemoglobin in the blood, hematocrit - the percentage of the blood made up of red blood cells, and the red blood cell indices (describes the average size and hemoglobin content of red blood cells).

Below, we'll review definitions, define ranges, present possible causes of imbalance, and provide supplement recommendations to optimize health.

WHITE BLOOD CELL (WBC) COUNT AND DIFFERENTIAL

White blood cell count measures the total number of white blood cells in a certain volume of blood. Since WBCs kill bacteria, this count is a measure of the body's response to infection and of the health of the overall immune system.

Here are the ranges used to observe WBC count:

Clinical Adult Range: 4,500-11,000cu.mm

Optimal Adult Range: 5,000-8,000cu.mm

Red Flag Range <3,000cu.mm or >13,000cu.mm

Some common causes of WBC increase include: active infections, leukemia, and childhood diseases (measles, mumps, chicken-pox, rubella, etc.)

Some common causes of WBC decrease include: chronic viral or bacterial Infections and lupus (SLE)

Clinical Note:

- An increase or decrease in total WBC level in conjunction with a lymphocyte count of below 20 and an albumin level below 4.0 is a pattern that is frequently seen in a developing tumor

Nutrition Note:

- A decreased WBC level may indicate a need for Vitamin B12, B6, and folic acid

NEUTROPHILS

Neutrophils are the most abundant type of white blood cells. They're the first responders at injury sites and play an important role in fighting infection and repairing tissue. They block, disable, and consume unwelcome pathogens.

These cells are most often elevated when there's an acute infection involved. An acute infection usually appears suddenly, is considered severe, and may be long or short-lived.

Here are the ranges used to observe neutrophil count:

Clinical Adult Range: 35-65 percent of total WBC

Optimal Adult Range: 40-60 percent of total WBC

Red Flag Range <30 percent of total WBC or >80 percent of total WBC

Common causes for neutrophil increase and decrease are the same as for general white blood cell count -

Some common causes of neutrophil increase include: active infections, leukemia, and childhood diseases (measles, mumps, chicken-pox, rubella, etc.)

Some common causes of neutrophil decrease include: chronic viral or bacterial Infections, lupus (SLE)

MONOCYTES

Monocytes are the largest of the white blood cells and are a key player in immune protection. They help to fight bacteria, viruses, and other infections in the body, and there is an elevated count of monocytes when bacterial and protozoal infections are present in the body.

Here are the ranges used to observe monocyte count:

Clinical Adult Range: 0-10% of total WBC

Optimal Adult Range: less than 7% of total WBC

Red Flag Range: >15 percent of total WBC

Some common causes of monocyte increase include: bacterial and parasitic infections, prostate hypertrophy, ovarian and uterine dysfunction

Some common causes of monocyte decrease include: a high corticosteroid dose

Clinical Note:

- An increase in monocyte level with an increase in basophils and a mild increase in eosinophils may indicate intestinal parasites

LYMPHOCYTES

Lymphocytes are an extremely important part of the immune response. They act as memory cells to remember previous immune breaches and help the body react more quickly to future attacks, and also scan cells in the body and kill the ones that have "gone bad" – for example, if they have been infected with foreign pathogens, or if they have become cancerous.

Here are the ranges used to observe lymphocyte count:

Clinical Adult Range: 20-40% of total WBC

Optimal Adult Range: 25-40% of total WBC

Red Flag Range: <20 percent of total WBC or >55 percent of total WBC

Some common causes of lymphocyte increase include: chronic viral or bacterial infection, autoimmune disease, childhood diseases (measles, mumps, chicken-pox, rubella, etc.), HIV, hepatitis, certain blood cancers

Some common causes of lymphocyte decrease include: Active infections, severe stress

Clinical Note:

- A viral infection may be present when lymphocytes increase to a point that either equals or exceeds your neutrophil level

EOSINOPHILS

Eosinophils help fight disease, and are often linked with allergic conditions, skin diseases, and parasitic diseases. They often moved to areas of the body that have become inflamed and "clean" house. Eosinophils also kill harmful invader cells, particularly of the bacterial and parasitic type.

Here are the ranges used to observe eosinophil count:

Clinical Adult Range: 0-7% of total WBC

Optimal Adult Range: 0-3% of total WBC

Red Flag Range <20 percent of total WBC or >55 percent of total WBC

Some common causes of eosinophil increase include: allergic conditions (asthma), food sensitivities, parasitic infection

BASOPHILS

Basophils are extremely important to immune system function. Like other types of white blood cells, they help fight infection and foreign invaders to the body. They contain both an anticoagulant and a histamine that helps sustain and increase blood flow to tissues.

Here are the ranges used to observe basophil count:

Clinical Adult Range: 0-2% of total WBC

Optimal Adult Range: 0-1% of total WBC

Red Flag Range <5 percent of total WBC

Some common causes of basophil increase include: Inflammation, childhood diseases (measles, mumps, chickenpox, rubella, etc.), acute trauma and parasites

Clinical Notes:

- If you have symptoms of inflammation in the absence of trauma, you should ask your doctor to order a C-Reactive Protein and/or Erythrocyte Sedimentation Rate test

- If basophils are increased with no sign of inflammation, consider asking your doctor to order a comprehensive stool and digestive test to rule out intestinal parasites

Supplement Recommendations

The following supplements can help support your white blood cells and overall immune function in your system:

- Vitamin D
- Vitamin C
- Zinc
- Elderberry
- Astragalus

RED BLOOD CELLS

Another important component of the CBC Panel is the Red Blood Cell (RBC) count. Red blood cells are made in the spleen and reveal the oxygen-carrying ability of the blood. This count is often used with other information to determine whether someone might be anemic. If your RBC levels are not normal, your doctor may order iron and/or ferritin tests.

Here are the ranges used to observe red blood cell count:

Clinical Adult Male Range: 4.60-6.0 million cu/mm

Optimal Adult Male Range: 4.20-4.90 million cu/mm

Red Flag Range for Men <3.90 or >6.00 million cu/mm

Clinical Adult Female Range: 3.90-5.50 million cu/mm

Optimal Adult Female Range: 3.90-4.50 million cu/mm

Red Flag Range for Women <3.50 or >5.00 million cu/mm

Some common causes of RBC increase include: polycythemia, dehydration, respiratory distress (asthma, emphysema)

Some common causes of RBC decrease include: iron deficiency anemia, internal bleeding

Nutrition Note:

- Low levels of RB indicate a need for B12, B6, and folic acid

HEMATOCRIT

This piece of the CBC panel defines the measurement of the percentage of red blood cells in whole blood. It is an important determinant of anemia (decreased), dehydration (elevated) or possible overhydration (decreased). If your hematocrit levels are not normal, your doctor may order a ferritin test.

Here are the ranges used to observe hematocrit:

Clinical Adult Male Range: 40.0-52.0 percent

Optimal Adult Male Range: 40.0-48.0 percent

Clinical Adult Female Range: 36.0-47.0 percent

Optimal Adult Female Range: 37.0-44.0 percent

Red Flag Range <32.0 or >55 percent

Some common causes of hematocrit increase include: polycythemia, dehydration, emphysema, asthma

Some common causes of hematocrit decrease include: anemia, internal bleeding, digestive inflammation

Clinical Notes:

- If iron, hemoglobin, and hematocrit levels are all low, you may have iron anemia
- If MCT, hematocrit, and iron levels are all low (check AST too!), you may have Vitamin B6 anemia
- If hematocrit, MCH, MCV, and iron levels are low, you may have Vitamin B12/folic acid anemia

HEMOGLOBIN

A hemoglobin test is used to measure the level of hemoglobin in your blood. Hemoglobin lives in your red blood cells, and is the transport vehicle of choice for oxygen and carbon dioxide in the blood. It's made up of a group of amino acids called "globin" and "heme," or iron, which allows it to bind to oxygen.

Hemoglobin tests are important because they can detect anemia or malabsorption due to poor nutrition and/or other factors.

Here are the ranges used to observe hemoglobin levels:

Clinical Adult Male Range: 13.5-18.0g/dL

Optimal Adult Male Range: 14.0-15.0g/dL

Clinical Adult Female Range: 12.5-16.0g/dL

Optimal Adult Female Range: 13.5-14.5g/dL

Red Flag Range <10.0 or >17g/dL

Some common causes of hemoglobin increase include: polycythemia, dehydration, emphysema, asthma

Some common causes of hemoglobin decrease include: anemia, internal bleeding, digestive inflammation

Clinical Note:

- Consider having your doctor check your iron and ferritin levels if you hemoglobin level is low

Nutrition Note:

- A low level of hemoglobin may indicate the need for
  Vitamin B12, folic acid, and thiamine

RED BLOOD CELL INDICES

This part of the CBC test helps to diagnose anemia. The RBC indices include a platelet count and measurements for MCV and MCH – we'll review these definitions and ranges below.

Mean Corpuscular Volume (MCV) The MCV indicates the volume occupied by the average red blood cell. In other words, the MCV measures the average size of your red blood cells.

Here are the ranges used to observe MCV:

Clinical Adult Range: 81.0-99.0 cu.microns

Optimal Adult Range: 82.0-89.9 cu.microns

Red Flag Range <78.0 or >95.0 cu.microns

A common cause of MCV count increase is: vitamin B-12/folic acid anemia

Some common causes of MCV count decrease include: iron anemia, internal bleeding

Mean Corpuscular Hemoglobin (MCH) The MCH measures the average amount of hemoglobin in a single red blood cell

Here are the ranges used to observe MCH:

Clinical Adult Range: 26.0-33.0 micro-micro grams

Optimal Adult Range: 27.0-31.9 micro-micro grams

Red Flag Range <24.0 or >34.0 micro-micro grams

Some common Causes of MCH Count Increase: Vitamin B-12/Folic Acid Anemia

Common Causes of MCH Count Decrease: Iron anemia, internal bleeding

Clinical Notes for MVH and MCH :

- If your MCV level is greater than 89.9 cu.microns and your MCH level is greater than 31.9 micro-micro grams, you may have Vitamin B12 or folic acid anemia. You should consider asking your doctor to confirm this by testing your levels
- If iron and ferritin levels are normal and MCV, MCH, hemoglobin, and hematocrit levels are all decreased – your body may have a toxic metal burden

PLATELET COUNT

Platelets, also called thrombocytes, help blood clot in order to stop or prevent bleeding.

Clinical Adult Range: 150,000-450,000cu.mm

Optimal Adult Range: 200,000-300,000cu.mm

Red Flag Range <50,000 or >600,000cu.mm

Some common causes of platelet increase include: polycythemia, inflammatory arthritis, several types of anemia, arteriosclerosis, acute blood loss

Some common causes of platelet decrease include: leukemia, liver dysfunction

Clinical Note:

- Quinidine, heparin, gold salts, sulfas, and digitoxin are all drugs that have been found to lower platelet count

Nutrition Note:

- A low platelet level may be a sign of Vitamin B12, folic acid, selenium, and iron deficiency

Supplement Recommendations

The following supplements can help support your red blood cell health:

- Vitamin C
- Iron
- Betaine-HCL
- Bovine Liver
- Vitamin B12

IRON TESTS

An iron test determines the levels of iron circulating in your bloodstream. Iron is an essential element in the body that is very important to the health of red blood cells. If you'll remember from the previous section, iron is the integral part of our friend hemoglobin that allows it to take oxygen to and from where it needs to go.

In addition to testing iron level specifically, it is also helpful to test ferritin and the reticulocyte count. Your doctor may suggest iron tests to complement your CBC panel.

Below, we'll review definitions of each of the points measured, define ranges, share common causes of abnormal levels, and share any supplements that may be taken to help balance levels.

IRON TEST

Again, iron is an essential element in your body that allows hemoglobin to transfer oxygen. If the body is low in iron, all body cells, particularly muscles in adults and brain cells in children, do not function at the level they need to. If your iron is low, you should consider getting a ferritin test, especially if you are a female who still has menstrual cycles.

Here are the ranges used to observe iron levels:

Clinical Adult Range: 40-150ug/ml

Optimal Adult Range: 50-100ug/ml

Red Flag Range <25ug/ml or >200ug/ml

Some common causes of iron increase include: Hemochromatosis, liver dysfunction, iron therapy, pernicious and hemolytic anemia. An additional cause for iron increase is cooking with iron utensils or overuse of iron supplements.

Some common causes of iron decrease include: pathologic bleeding (especially in geriatric population) and iron deficiency anemia.

Clinical Note:

- An iron evaluation complete when paired with a ferritin test (see below)

Nutrition Note:

- An increased iron level with decreased hematocrit suggests intrinsic factor deficiency

FERRITIN TEST

Ferritin is a protein that lives inside your body's cells (mostly liver and immune system cells) and stores iron, releasing the precious element as needed. The ferritin test is considered the "gold standard" in documenting iron deficiency anemia. Levels below 25 indicate a need for iron.

Here are the ranges used to observe ferritin levels:

Clinical Male Adult Range: 33-236ng/mL

Optimal Male Adult Range: 20-200ng/mL

Clinical Female Adult Range (before menopause): 11-122ng/mL

Optimal Female Adult Range (before menopause): 10-110ng/mL

Clinical Female Adult Range (after menopause): 12-263ng/mL

Optimal Female Adult Range(after menopause): 20-200ng/mL

Red Flag Range <8ng/mL or >500ng/mL

Low levels below 25 indicate a need for iron. High levels may an inflammatory disorder, infections, rheumatoid arthritis, chronic kidney disease

Some common causes of ferritin increase include: iron overload and hemochromatosis. Additional causes include inflammation, infections, rheumatoid arthritis, and chronic kidney disease.

A common cause of ferritin decrease is: iron deficiency anemia

Clinical Notes:

- A ferritin level of greater than 1000 may be a sign of hemochromatosis
- Iron overload and/or hemochromatosis are silent and can result in cirrhosis of the liver, bacterial infections, dementia, arteriosclerosis, diabetes, and stroke

Nutrition Note:

- Doctors specializing in chelation have found a correlation with increased iron and arteriosclerosis

RETICULOCYTE COUNT TEST

Reticulocytes are immature red blood cells produced by the bone marrow and released into the blood. Reticulocytes could be considered "baby" red blood cells, and they take about 2 days to develop into fully mature red blood cells.

A reticulocyte count test is used to confirm chronic microscopic bleeding, as the count rises when there are high levels of blood loss or when red blood cells are destroyed prematurely. This test is also used to diagnose and determine if anemia is present.

Here are the ranges used to observe reticulocyte count:

Clinical Adult Range: 0.5-1.5%

Optimal Adult Range: same as clinical range

Red Flag Range >2.0%

A common causes of reticulocyte count increase is: internal bleeding

Some common causes of reticulocyte count decrease include: vitamin B12, B6, and folic acid anemia

Supplement Recommendations

The following supplements can help support the right balance of iron in your system:

- Vitamin C
- Iron
- Betaine-HCL
- Bovine Liver
- Vitamin 12

THE BASIC METABOLIC PANEL - BMP

A basic metabolic panel is a blood test that measures your sugar (glucose) level, electrolyte and fluid balance, and kidney function. Glucose is a type of sugar your body uses for energy. Electrolytes keep your body's fluids in balance. They also help keep your body working normally, assisting in important functions such as your heart rhythm, muscle contraction, and brain function.

The kidneys help keep the right balance of water, salts, and minerals in the blood. Kidneys also filter out waste and other unneeded substances from the blood.

If you take any medicines, such as diuretics for high blood pressure, your doctor may order a basic metabolic panel to see if the medicines are affecting your kidneys or your electrolytes. Your doctor also may order this panel as part of a regular health examination or to help diagnose a medical condition.

This panel measures the blood levels of blood urea nitrogen (BUN), calcium, carbon dioxide, chloride, creatinine, glucose, potassium, and sodium.

Below, we'll review definitions, define ranges, present possible causes of imbalance, and provide supplement recommendations to optimize health.

BLOOD UREA NITROGEN (BUN)

BUN is a waste product derived from protein breakdown in the liver. This measurement shows how much urea nitrogen is in your blood, which shows if your liver and kidneys are working properly.

Here are the ranges used to observe BUN levels:

Clinical Adult Range: 10-26 mg/dL

Optimal Adult Range: 13-18 mg/dL

Red Flag Range <5 or >50 mg/dL

Some common causes of BUN increase include: excessive protein intake, renal (kidney) disease or damage, gout, certain drugs, low fluid intake, intestinal bleeding, exercise, heart failure, decreased digestive enzyme production by the pancreas.

Some common causes of BUN decrease include: inadequate protein intake, malabsorption, liver damage, pregnancy

CREATININE

Creatinine is a waste product produced by muscles from the breakdown of the amino acid creatine. You might associate creatine as a weight-lifting supplement, but it's something that's found naturally in animal protein. The level of creatinine in your body is a reflection of the body's muscle mass. Elevated levels are generally reflective of kidney damage and need to be monitored very carefully.

Here are the ranges used to observe creatinine levels:

Clinical Adult Range: 0.7-1.5 mg/dL

Optimal Adult Range: 0.7-1.0 mg/dL

Red Flag Range >1.6 mg/dL

Some common causes of creatinine increase include: kidney problems and gout. Additional causes include uncontrolled diabetes, congestive heart failure, urinary tract infection, and dehydration.

A common cause of creatinine decrease is: amyotonia congenita

Clinical Notes:

- If creatinine level is 1.2 or higher in a male over the age of 40, prostate hypertrophy MUST be ruled out
- A creatinine level between 2-4 mg/dl may be an indicator of early kidney disease. It may indicate severe kidney disease if the creatinine level is between 4-35 mg/dl.

BUN/CREATININE RATIO

The ratio of BUN and creatinine ratio in your body are again, important indicators of whether your liver and kidneys are working properly.

Here are the ranges used to observe the BUN/Creatinine ratio:

Clinical Adult Range: 6-10

Optimal Adult Range: 10-20

Red Flag Range <5 or >30

Some common causes of BUN/Creatinine ratio increase include: catabolic states, dehydration, circulatory failure leading to a fall in renal (kidney) blood flow, congestive heart failure, acute and chronic kidney failure, urinary tract obstruction, enlargement of the prostate, a high protein diet

Some common causes of BUN/Creatinine ratio decrease include: overhydration, low protein/high carb diet

Clinical Notes:

- Decreased BUN levels less than 8 with a decreased urinary specific gravity may indicate posterior pituitary dysfunction
- Increased BUN levels above 25 usually indicates kidney disease. However, if creatinine is not above 1.1, then kidney disease may not be the problem. Instead, consider anterior pituitary dysfunction, dehydration, or hypochlorhydria.

Nutrition Note:

- Increased BUN levels may indicate a boron deficiency

CALCIUM

Calcium is the most abundant mineral in the body. It is involved in bone metabolism, protein absorption, fat transfer, muscular contraction, transmission of nerve impulses, blood clotting, and heart function. It is highly sensitive to elements such as magnesium, iron, and phosphorous as well as hormonal activity, vitamin D levels, CO2 levels and many drugs.

Diet, or even the presence of calcium in the diet has a lot to do with "calcium balance" - how much calcium you take in and how much you lose from your body. In addition, poor intestinal fat absorption may be suspected with low levels of calcium, bilirubin, and phosphorus.

Here are the ranges used to observe calcium levels:

Clinical Adult Range: 8.5-10.8

Optimal Adult Range: 9.7-10.1

Red Flag Range <7.0 mg/dL or >12.0 mg/dL

A common cause of calcium increase is: hyperparathyroidism. Additional causes of calcium increase may include: tumor of the thyroid, hypervitaminosis (excess Vitamin D), multiple myeloma, neurofibromatosis, osteoporosis, ovarian hypo-function, adrenal hypo-function

Some common causes of calcium decrease may include: hypoparathyroidism, pregnancy, hypochlorhydria, kidney dysfunction. Additional causes of calcium decrease may include a Vitamin D deficiency, diarrhea, celiac disease, lacking protein in the diet

Clinical Notes:

- Protein levels are influenced by calcium levels. Calcium goes up with increased protein and goes down with decreased protein.
- Poor intestinal fat absorption may be suspected with low levels of calcium, bilirubin, and phosphorus.
- If calcium levels are either above or below normal, abnormal circadian rhythm should be a primary consideration

Nutrition Note:

- Pancreatic enzyme deficiency may be suspected with low levels of calcium, triglycerides, and increased levels of LDH

CO2 LEVEL

Your CO2 level is related to the respiratory exchange of carbon dioxide in the lungs and is part of the body's buffering system. Generally, when used with other electrolytes, carbon dioxide levels indicate pH or acid/alkaline balance in the tissues.

CO2 is one of the most important things we measure. Most people have too much acid in their body. As you might know, it's very difficult to grow plants in soil where the pH is incorrect. Our blood is similar to soil in many respects and it will be difficult to be healthy if our body's pH is not well balanced.

Here are the ranges used to observe CO_2 levels:

Clinical Adult Range: 24-32mmol/L

Optimal Adult Range: 26-30mmol/L

Red Flag Range <18mmol/L or >38mmol/L

Some common causes of CO_2 increase include: alkalosis, hypochlorhydria. Other causes of CO_2 increase may include acute vomiting, fever, adrenal hyperfunction, and emphysema.

A common cause of CO_2 decrease is: acidosis. Other causes of CO_2 decrease may include diabetes, sleep apnea, and severe diarrhea.

Clinical Note:

- If CO_2 level is above 32 mmol/L, you should ask your doctor to conduct a Pulmonary Function Test

Nutrition Note:

- Low levels of CO_2 may indicate a need for thiamine (Vitamin B1)

CHLORIDE

Chloride is an electrolyte controlled by the kidneys and levels may sometimes be affected by diet. This is an electrolyte involved in maintaining acid-base balance and helps to regulate blood volume and artery pressure.

Here are the ranges used to observe chloride levels:

Clinical Adult Range: 96-110 mmol/L

Optimal Adult Range: 100-106 mmol/L

Red Flag Range <90 or >115 mmol/L

Some common causes of chloride increase include: kidney problems, metabolic acidosis, too much water crossing the cell membrane. Other causes may include hyperventilation, anemia, prostate problems, excess intake of salt, and dehydration.

Some common causes of chloride decrease include: kidney problems, metabolic alkalosis, hypochlorhydria (too little acid in the stomach). Other causes may include diabetes, pneumonia, and intestinal obstruction.

Clinical Notes:

- Hypochlorhydria is a suspect if chloride is below 100, total globulin is less than 2.4, and phosphorus is less than 3.0
- Chloride is required for the production of HCL by the chief cells of the stomach

GLUCOSE

Glucose is the main sugar found in your blood and it is the chief source of energy for all living organisms. A common phrase used to describe the glucose level in the body is "blood sugar."

Some important things to note in this test are that a level greater than 105 in someone who has fasted for 12 hours suggests a diabetic tendency. If this level is elevated even in a non-fasting setting one must be concerned that there is a risk for developing diabetes. This is an incredibly powerful test and can predict diabetes ten years or more before one develops the strict definition of diabetes which is levels greater than 120.

Here are the ranges used to observe glucose levels:

Clinical Adult Range: 70-115 mg/dL

Optimal Adult Range: 85-100 mg/dL

Red Flag Range <50 or >250 mg/dL

Some common causes of glucose increase include: diabetes, poor carbohydrate utilization, syndrome X.

A common cause of glucose decrease is: fasting hypo-glycemia. Other causes may include liver damage and Addison's disease.

Clinical Notes:

- LDH will frequently be decreased or in the low normal with fasting hypoglycemia. However, LDH will almost always be decreased with reactive hypoglycemia.
- A glycohemoglobin (HGC A1C) test may be ordered when serum glucose values are above 160, and to help monitor diabetics under therapy.

Nutrition Note:

- Thiamine deficiency has been linked to an increase in glucose levels.

POTASSIUM

This is an element that is found primarily inside the cells of the body. It is both a mineral and an electrolyte and assists with essential functions in the body – in this case, helping your nervous system to function smoothly as well as assisting muscles to contract properly. Low potassium levels can cause muscle weakness and heart problems.

Here are the ranges used to observe potassium levels:

Clinical Adult Range: 3.5-5.0

Optimal Adult Range: 4.0-4.6

Red Flag Range <3.0 or >6.0 mmol/L

Some common causes of potassium increase include: adrenal hypofunction, cortisol resistance, acidosis, ongoing tissue destruction

Some common causes of potassium decrease include: severe diarrhea, alcoholism, excessive use of water pills, kidney problems, adrenal hyperfunction

Nutrition Note:

- Excessive licorice consumption has been linked to lower potassium levels.

SODIUM

This element plays an important role in salt and water balance in your body that plays an important role for muscle and nerve function and regulating blood pressure levels.

Here are the ranges used to observe sodium levels:

Clinical Adult Range: 135-145

Optimal Adult Range: 140-144

Red Flag Range <125 or >155 mmol/L

Some common causes of sodium increase include: too much salt intake, nephritis (kidney problems), dehydration, hypercorticoadrenalism (increased adrenal function)

Some common causes of sodium decrease include: too much water intake, heart failure, kidney failure, reduced kidney filtration, diarrhea, vomiting, Addison's disease, adrenal hypo-function

Clinical Note:

- Water softeners may be a cause of increased sodium levels.

MAGNESIUM

Magnesium is a very important element found in the arteries, heart, bone, muscles, nerves, and teeth. It is responsible for a multitude of bodily functions. Among other things, It helps muscles and nerves function well, regulates blood pressure, and supports the immune system. It also helps regulate glucose and insulin levels in the body.

Magnesium is one of the most common deficiencies in society today. People who tend to have spasticity, stiffness in the morning, anxiety, depression, restless leg, or an overall sense of tension, may have a magnesium deficiency.

Here are the ranges used to observe magnesium levels:

Clinical Adult Range: 1.7-2.4

Optimal Adult Range: 2.2-2.6

Red Flag Range <1.2 mg/dL

A common cause of magnesium increase is: kidney problems

Some common symptoms of magnesium deficiency include: anxiety, aching muscles, disorientation, low body temperature, easily angered, hyperactivity, insomnia, muscle tremors, nervousness, rapid pulse, sensitivity to noise and loud sounds, epilepsy

Clinical Notes:

- Magnesium should be evaluated on all patients suffering with heart disease.
- Those suffering from fibromyalgia may have a low serum magnesium accompanied with a low CO_2 level and an increased anion gap
- If your magnesium is less than 2.0, it is strongly recommended to have an erythrocyte magnesium test or a magnesium loading test

Nutrition/Lifestyle Notes:

- Excessive use of antacids containing magnesium may increase magnesium levels
- Blue light from electronic devices will actually deplete magnesium!

PHOSPHORUS

Phosphorus is closely associated with calcium in bone development. In fact, calcium *needs* phosphorus to strengthen teeth and bones – it's the quiet mineral working behind the scenes to help calcium do its job. While most phosphorus is found in the skeletal system, in the blood, phosphorus is an important player in the proper function of muscles and nerves.

Blood must be drawn carefully with this test, as improper handling can create a false increase in the results.

Therefore most of the phosphate in the body is found in the bones. But the phosphorus level in the blood is very important for muscle and nerve function. Very low levels of phosphorus in the blood can be associated with starvation or malnutrition and this can lead to muscle weakness. High levels in the blood are usually associated with kidney disease. However the blood must be drawn carefully as improper handling may falsely increase the reading.

Here are the ranges used to observe phosphorus levels:

Clinical Adult Range: 2.5-4.5

Optimal Adult Range: 3.2-3.9

Red Flag Range <2.0 mg/dL or >5.0 mg/dL

Some common causes of phosphorus increase include: parathyroid dysfunction, kidney disease, excessive phosphoric acid in soft drinks. Additional causes include bone tumors, diabetes, and excess intake of Vitamin D.

Some common causes of phosphorus decrease include: Parathyroid hyperfunction, osteomalacia, and rickets. Additional causes include diabetes, malnutrition/starvation, and liver dysfunction.

Clinical Notes:

- Vitamin D deficiency may be present if there are low levels of calcium and phosphorus with increased levels of alkaline phosphorus
- Phosphorus is a general indicator of digestive function. Consider hypochlorhydria when phosphorus level is below 3.0 and total globulin level is greater than 3.0 or less than 2.4
- Children will have an increase in phosphorus level due to normal bone growth. People with any fractures will also have an increased phosphorus level.

Nutrition Note:

- Phosphorus level is frequently decreased with diets high in refined sugars

Supplement Recommendations

The following supplements can help optimize your metabolic support functions:

- Magnesium Chelate
- Calcium
- Inositol
- Rhodiola
- Ashwagandha

THE LIPID (FATS) PANEL

A lipid panel is a test used to measure different fats and fatty substances in your body. Fat sort of has a bad reputation, but in proper levels in the body, it carries out some essential functions. They provide the body with energy and warmth, and also produce important hormones and help with nutrient absorption. Fat also provides a valuable cushion for our internal organs. We need to make sure our fat is optimized and doing its job!

A standard lipid panel will measure your total cholesterol level, HDL cholesterol level, LDL cholesterol level, and triglyceride level. Imbalances in these lipids can be an indicator of serious disease such as heart attack, stroke, and disease of the arteries.

A doctor may order this test to determine whether you are at risk for one of the life-threatening illnesses listed above, or to provide a diagnosis for such a disease.

Below, we'll review definitions of each of the points measured, define ranges, share common causes of abnormal levels, and share supplements that may be taken to help balance levels.

TOTAL CHOLESTEROL LEVEL

Cholesterol is a group of fats vital to cell membranes, nerve fibers and bile salts, and a necessary precursor for the sex hormones. Cholesterol values below 140 is a sign of a serious issue.

Here are the ranges used to observe cholesterol levels:

Clinical Adult Range: 120-200mg/dL

Optimal Adult Range: 150-180mg/dL

Red Flag Range <50mg/dL or >400mg/dL

Some common causes of cholesterol increase include: diet high in carbs and sugars, early stages of diabetes, fatty liver, arteriosclerosis, hypothyroidism. Additional causes include multiple sclerosis and pregnancy.

Some common causes of cholesterol decrease include: a low-fat diet, malabsorption, anemia, carbohydrate sensitivity, liver dysfunction, chemical/heavy metal overload, hyperthyroidism, viral hepatitis, free radical pathology

Clinical Notes:

- A cholesterol level below 130 is considered an ominous sign
- If cholesterol level is above 200 with an AST level below 10, suspect liver congestion/fatty liver

Nutrition Note:

- Increased cholesterol levels have been found to be lowered by the amino acid methionine

HDL (HIGH DENSITY LIPOPROTEIN) CHOLESTEROL

You may have heard about the "good" and "bad" cholesterol. HDL is the "good" cholesterol, and essential fat that is the densest of the cholesterol particles. HDL offers protection against chronic heart disease also helps remove cholesterol from the peripheral tissues and transports it back to the liver, where it is broken down and removed from the body.

A high level of HDL is an indication of a healthy metabolic system if there is no sign of liver disease or intoxication.

Here are the ranges used to observe HDL cholesterol levels:

Clinical Adult Males Range: >50mg/dL

Optimal Adult Male Range: >55mg/dL

Clinical Adult Female Range: >55mg/dL

Optimal Adult Female Range: >60mg/dL

Red Flag Range <35mg/dL

Some common causes of HDL cholesterol decrease include: arteriosclerosis (hardening of the arteries), diabetes, Syndrome X. Additional causes of HDL cholesterol decrease include cigarette smoking and taking steroids and beta-blockers.

Clinical Note:

- If HDL level is decreased, triglycerides are greater than 50% of the cholesterol value, LDL level is increased, and uric acid is increased – this combination rules out arteriosclerosis

Nutrition Note:

- A diet high in refined carbohydrates, a lack of exercise, and genetic predisposition have been shown to lower HDL levels.

LDL (LOW DENSITY LIPOPROTEIN) CHOLESTEROL

LDL cholesterol would be what some refer to as the "bad" cholesterol. It has been known to gather along the walls of blood vessels, increasing the chances of disease like heart attack or stroke.

Here are the ranges used to observe LDL cholesterol levels:

Clinical Adult Range: <130mg/dL

Optimal Adult Range: <120mg/dL

Red Flag Range >180mg/dL

Some common causes of LDL cholesterol increase include: arteriosclerosis (hardening of the arteries), diabetes, Syndrome X

TOTAL CHOLESTEROL/HDL RATIO

This ratio is an important marker for cardiovascular health. A ratio <4.0 is considered adequate. A ratio <3.1 is ideal. A higher ratio can mean increased risks of heart disease.

TRIGLYCERIDES

Triglycerides are a type of fat found in your blood, and is also the type of fat stored in your fat cells. They are usually stored until used as fuel by the body or as an energy source for metabolism.

Here are the ranges used to observe triglyceride levels:

Clinical Adult Range: 50-150mg/dL

Optimal Adult Range: 70-110mg/dL

Red Flag Range <35mg/dL or >350mg/dL

Some common causes of triglyceride increase include: hyperlipidemia, diabetes, and alcoholism. Additional causes include hypothyroidism and early stages of fatty liver.

Some common causes of triglyceride decrease include: chemical/heavy metal overload, liver dysfunction, hyperthyroidism

Clinical Note:

- Resistive exercise training has been found to be effective in lowering elevated triglycerides

∿

Supplement Recommendations

Because cholesterol is produced and regulated in large part by the liver, I recommend following a liver detox protocol to assist with optimizing fatty metabolism support in your system.

THE LIVER PANEL

The liver is the large, underrated workhorse of our bodily system. Officially classified as a gland, not only does it break down fat and extra carbs into energy forms we can save for later, it is a major contributor in the detoxification and immunity game.

Our livers also produce bile to help the small intestine break down food, store lots of vitamins and minerals, and helps filter our blood. If you haven't already, please say thank you to your liver today.

The liver panel (or liver function panel) is a test that is conducted to see, well, how the liver is doing. It measures for protein and enzyme levels – protein measurements include a total protein overview, albumin, globulin, and an albumin/globulin (A/G) ratio. Enzymes measured include alkaline phosphatase, ALT, AST, and GGT.

Your doctor may order a liver panel to assess general health, or if you have symptoms of liver disease. A liver panel may also be ordered if you have diabetes, a high triglyceride level, anemia, or high blood pressure.

Below, we'll review definitions of each of the points measured, define ranges, share common causes of abnormal levels, and share any supplements that may be taken to help balance levels.

PROTEINS

TOTAL PROTEIN

Total Protein: This is a measure of the total amount of protein in your blood. Total protein is the combination of albumin and total globulin and is affected by the albumin and total globulin. A low or high total protein does not indicate a specific disease, but it does indicate that some additional tests may be required to determine if there is a problem.

Here are the ranges used to observe total protein levels:

Clinical Adult Range: 6.0-8.5g/dL

Optimal Adult Range: 7.1-7.6g/dL

Red Flag Range <5.9g/dL or > 8.5g/dL

Some common causes of protein increase include: dehydration, "early" carcinoma, multiple myeloma (should be correlated with serum protein electrophoresis). Additional causes may include diabetes and rheumatoid arthritis.

Some common causes of protein decrease include: protein malnutrition and digestive inflammation.

Nutrition Notes:

- If protein and calcium are found to be on the low side of the optimal range, there may be poor protein absorption
- Decreased levels of protein, cholesterol and ALT may indicate fatty liver congestion

ALBUMIN

Albumin is the most abundant protein in the blood. It is made in the liver and is an antioxidant that protects your tissues from free radicals. It binds waste products, toxins and dangerous drugs that might damage the body. It is also a major buffer in the body and plays a role in controlling the precise amount of water in our tissues. It serves to transport vitamins, minerals and hormones.

Here are the ranges used to observe albumin levels:

Clinical Adult Range: 3.0-5.5

Optimal Adult Range: 4.0-4.4

Red Flag Range <4.0 g/dL

A common cause of albumin increase is: dehydration. Additional causes may include thyroid and adrenal hypo-function.

A common causes of albumin decrease is: liver disease. Additional causes are a poor diet, vitamin deficiencies, diarrhea, fever, infection, kidney disease, gall bladder disease, and multiple sclerosis.

Clinical Notes:

- An albumin level of 3.5 or below with a lymphocyte count of 1500 or less is one of the Four Ominous Signs
- An albumin level of higher than 2.7 is one of the Four Ominous Signs

Nutrition Note:

- A low albumin level combined with a low phosphorus level may indicate digestive inflammation

GLOBULIN

Globulins have many diverse functions, including being a carrier of hormones, lipids, metals, and antibodies. They are part of immune system function and also assist the body with blood clotting and fighting infection.

Here are the ranges used to observe globulin levels:

Clinical Adult Range: 2.0-4.0

Optimal Adult Range: 2.8-3.5

Red Flag Range <2.0 g/dL or >3.5 g/100ml

Some common causes of globulin increase include: hypochlorhydria and liver disease/infection. Additional causes include chronic infection, rheumatoid arthritis, myelomas, and lupus.

Some common causes of globulin decrease include: anemia and hemorrhage. Additional causes included compromise of the immune system, poor dietary habits, malabsorption, and liver and kidney disease.

Clinical Notes:

- Anytime the total globulin level is less than 2.0 or greater than 3.5, a serum protein electrophoresis test should be done.

A/G (ALBUMIN/GLOBULIN) RATIO

The A/G ratio shows the amount of albumin you have in your system compared with globulin, and can be an important indicator of disease. An A/G ratio of less than 1.0 is considered a sign of a serious condition.

Here are the ranges used to observe the A/G ratio:

Clinical Adult Range: 1.1-2.5

Optimal Adult Range: 1.2-1.5

Red Flag Range <1.0

Some causes of a low, red-flagged ratio include ulcerative colitis, burns, kidney disease, cirrhosis, multiple myeloma.

Clinical Note:

- An A/G ratio of less than 1.0 is one of the Four Ominous Signs

Nutrition Note:

- An elevated A/G ratio with elevated protein and cholesterol may indicate too much protein consumption

ENZYMES

ALKALINE PHOSPHATASE

Alkaline phosphatase is an enzyme that is found in all body tissue, but the most important sites are bone, liver, bile ducts and the gut. Growing children, because of bone growth, normally have a higher level of this enzyme than adults do.

Here are the ranges used to observe alkaline phosphatase levels:

Clinical Adult Range: 30-115

Optimal Adult Range: 60-80

Red Flag Range <30U/L or >Laboratory range

Some common causes of alkaline phosphatase increase include: bone, liver, or bile duct disease; certain drug use, rheumatoid arthritis. Additional causes include excess ingestion of Vitamin D, cirrhosis of the liver, alcoholism, and jaundice.

Some common causes of alkaline phosphatase decrease include: Anemia, Hypothyroidism, and celiac disease. Additional causes include adrenal hypofunction, protein or zinc or Vitamin C deficiency, and malnutrition.

Clinical Notes:

- If you have a significant increase in alkaline

phosphatase, you should ask your doctor for an ALP
isoenzyme test

- It is considered "normal" for the alkaline phosphatase
level to be elevated in children under 18 and people
with bone fractures

Nutrition Note:

- An alkaline phosphatase level below 70 u/l may
indicate a zinc deficiency.

ALANINE AMINOTRANSFERASE (ALT)

ALT (formerly known as SGPT) is a type of enzyme that is
primarily found in the liver and also in the kidneys, heart, and
skeletal system. Enzymes in the liver assist with protein breakdown and absorption. When there is damage or inflammation
to the liver, ALT may be released into the blood stream and can
be an indicator of disease.

Here are the ranges used to observe ALT levels:

Clinical Adult Range: 0-41

Optimal Adult Range: 18-26

Red Flag Range >100 U/L

Some common causes of ALT increase include: acute hepatitis, cirrhosis of liver, and mononucleosis. Additional causes include overuse of alcohol, liver and bile duct disease, and diabetes.

ASPARTATE AMINOTRANSFERASE (AST)

AST (formerly known as SGOT) is another enzyme found in the heart, skeletal muscles, brain, liver and kidneys. AST levels in the body are generally quite low and will increase when damage or inflammation occur in the liver and other organs and tissues.

Here are the ranges used to observe AST levels:

Clinical Adult Range: 0-41

Optimal Adult Range: 18-26

Red Flag Range >100 U/L

Some common causes of AST increase include: myocardial infarction, pulmonary embolism, congestive heart failure, myocarditis. Additional causes include hepatitis, liver disease, pancreatitis.

Clinical Notes for ALT and AST:

- In acute congestive heart failure and/or myocardial infarction, the AST and ALT levels will significantly increase. However, these values will slowly return to normal. AST level returns to normal more slowly and ALT level.

- ALT values are greater than AST in liver obstruction and toxic hepatitis.
- AST values are greater than ALT in cirrhosis of the liver, liver neoplasms, and jaundice

Nutrition Note:

- Low levels of AST and ALT may indicate a Vitamin B6 deficiency.

GAMMA-GLUTAMYL TRANSFERASE (GGT)

GGT is another enzyme found mainly in the liver, but also in the gallbladder, spleen, pancreas, and kidneys. It functions as a transporter of amino acids to other cells, and also plays the important job of assisting the liver in metabolizing drugs and other toxins. An increase in GGT levels may be an indicator of damage and disease in the liver and other organs.

Here are the ranges used to observe GGT levels:

Clinical Adult Range: 0-55U/L

Optimal Adult Range: 10-30U/L

Red Flag Range >90U/L

Some common causes of GGT increase include: alcoholism, bile duct obstruction, and inflammation of the bile duct and gallbladder. Additional causes include excess magnesium in the system, infection, hepatitis, and mononucleosis.

A possible cause of GGT decrease is: a vitamin B6 deficiency.

Clinical Notes:

- If GGT level is greater than 150 u/l with a bilirubin level of over 2.8 mg/dL, there is a high chance of biliary obstruction. You should seek medical attention immediately.
- If GGT values are 5x higher than the clinical range, you should suspect pancreatitis
- Food and allergy sensitivity are a common finding with biliary dysfunction

Supplement Recommendations

To provide support to your liver and balance the functions of the liver in your body, I recommend following a liver detox protocol.

THE THYROID PANEL

A thyroid panel is a blood test to determine the overall state of how your thyroid is functioning. Your thyroid is a gland on the front of your neck, and it's responsible for regulating metabolism and growth in your body. Every single cell in your body relies on the thyroid to regulate its metabolism. It also plays a huge part in helping with hormonal balance. When your thyroid isn't working properly, a variety of health issues can crop up.

Your thyroid is very important to overall wellness, and it's important to determine if it's healthy and working properly – and the best way to do that is to do the thyroid panel.

The thyroid panel test will measure the following points of thyroid function:

- Triiodothyronine (T3)
- Thyroxine (T4)
- T7
- T3 Uptake
- Thyroid Stimulating Hormone (TSH)

Below, we'll review definitions of each of the points measured, define ranges, share common causes of abnormal levels, and share any supplements that may be taken to help balance levels.

TRIIODOTHYRONINE (T3)

T3 is one of the important thyroid hormones – together with T4, they help to regulate metabolism and weight, digestive function, brain health, and musculoskeletal health. T3 can be found both bound to proteins in the body and traveling "freely," though most are bound to proteins. The term total T3 describes the total of both protein-bound and free T3.

Here are the ranges used to observe T3 levels:

Clinical Adult Range: 22-33%

Optimal Adult Range: 26-30%

A common cause of T3 increase is: hyperthyroidism

A common cause of T3 decrease is: hypothyroidism

THYROXINE/TETRAIODOTHYRONINE (T4)

T4 is the major hormone secreted by the thyroid gland. Together with T3, they help to regulate metabolism and weight, digestive function, brain health, and musculoskeletal health. T4 can be found both bound to other proteins in the body and traveling "freely," though most are bound to proteins. The term total T4 describes the total of both protein-bound and free T4.

Here are the ranges used to observe T4 levels:

Clinical Adult Range: 4.0-12.0mcg/dL

Optimal Adult Range: 7.0-8.5mcg/dL

A common cause of T4 increase is: hyperthyroidism

Some common causes of T4 decrease are: hypothyroidism and anterior pituitary hypo- function

FTI-FREE THYROXINE INDEX (T7)

T7 is an estimate, calculated by multiplying the total T4 level and the T3 uptake described below. It helps clarify test results when there is an abnormal level of binding proteins.

Clinical Adult Range: 4.0-12.0mcg/dL

Optimal Adult Range: 7.0-8.5mcg/dL

Some common causes of T7increase are: see T3 uptake description below

Some common causes of T7 decrease are: See T3 uptake description below

T3 RESIN UPTAKE (T3 UPTAKE OR T3RU)

Most protein-bound T3 and T4 in your body are bound to the specific protein thyroxine-binding globulin, or TBG. You can think of TBG as a little thyroid hormone taxi that helps shuttle T3 and T4 around the bloodstream. The T3 uptake is used to estimate how much TBG is in your blood, and also how much T3 and T4 are floating protein-free.

Here are the ranges used to observe T3 uptake levels:

Clinical Adult Range: 22-36%

Optimal Adult Range: 27-37%

Red Flag Range <20 percent of uptake or >39 percent of uptake

A common cause of T3 uptake increase is: thyroid hyperfunction. Additional causes include kidney dysfunction, salicylates toxicity, and protein malnutrition.

A common cause of T3 uptake decrease is: thyroid hypofunction

THYROID STIMULATING HORMONE (TSH)

TSH is produced in the pituitary gland and is the hormone that tells the thyroid to make hormones and send them off into the body. Testing levels for TSH used to confirm or rule out suspected hypothyroidism when T3, T4, and T7 are normal, but other signs point to hypothyroidism.

Here are the ranges used to observe TSH levels:

Clinical Adult Range: 0.4-4.4mlU/L

Optimal Adult Range: 2.0-4.0mlU/L

Red Flag Range <0.3mlU/L or >10.0mlU/L

A common cause of TSH increase is: thyroid hypo-function.

Clinical Notes:

- Underarm temperature will frequently be below 97.8 degrees Fahrenheit with thyroid hypofunction. If you suspect you may have issues in this area, you should take your underarm temperature for 10 minutes before leaving bed in the morning for five days in a row and average your number. This low underarm temperature is also common with adrenal stress, thiamine deficiency, and diets that lack essential fatty acids and protein.

TESTING FOR INFLAMMATORY
MARKERS

Inflammation is the body's innate response to injury or insult, including infection, trauma, surgery, burns, and cancer. Certain proteins are released into the bloodstream during inflammation; if their concentrations increase or decrease by at least 25%, they can be used as systemic inflammatory markers.

Although there are many inflammatory markers, also known as acute phase reactants, those most commonly measured in clinical practice (and discussed in this topic) are C-reactive protein (hsCRP), lactate dehydrogenase (LDH), and erythrocyte sedimentation rate (ESR).

Because these markers are nonspecific, the tests are not diagnostic for any particular condition, but they may help to identify a generalized inflammatory state along with other tests and aid in the differential diagnosis. In some diseases, serial measurements of CRP also may be of prognostic value.

Irregular values can commonly represent autoimmune issues, systemic inflammation, cardiac inflammation, and arthritic types of disorders.

C-REACTIVE PROTEIN (HSCRP)

hsCRP is a very sensitive version of CRP, a protein that is produced and released by the liver when there is inflammation in the body. A high level of hsCRP in the system can be an indicator of heart disease.

Here are the ranges used to observe hsCRP levels:

Clinical Adult Range: 1.0 - 3.0 mg/L

Optimal Adult Range: <1.0 mg/L

Red Flag Range: >3.0 mg/L

Some common causes of hsCRP increase include: cardiovascular disease, periodontal disease, acute illness (cold, flu, or infection), chronic illness (bronchitis or COPD), and autoimmune disorders

LACTATE DEHYDROGENASE (LDH) TEST

LDH is an enzyme that makes energy and is found in almost every cell in the body, but most numerously in the heart, liver, muscles, kidney, lungs, and red blood cells. When there is cell damage, this enzyme is released into blood plasma. Slightly elevated levels in the blood are common and usually are not a sign of disease, but more significantly elevated levels can signify issues.

Here are the ranges used to observe LDH levels:

Clinical Adult Range: 60-225U/L

Optimal Adult Range: 140-200U/L

Red Flag Range >250U/L

Some common causes of LDH increase include: liver & bile duct dysfunction, pulmonary embolism, hepatitis, myocardial infarction, tissue inflammation, tissue destruction, malignancy anywhere in the body and several types of anemias.

Clinical Notes:

- LDH level will frequently increase with low thyroid function and birth control usage

Nutrition Note:

- A decreased LDH level may indicate reactive hypoglycemia, and you should have your glucose levels checked.

ERYTHROCYTE SEDIMENTATION RATE (ESR) TEST

An ESR test measures how quickly red blood cells (erythrocytes) settle to the bottom of a blood sample. If the cells settle more quickly than normal, it can be a sign of inflammation in the body. This test documents helps to show if organic disease is really present in patients with vague symptoms and also helps to monitor chronic inflammatory conditions such as arthritis, vasculitis, or IBS.

Here are the ranges used to observe ESR:

Women under age 50 should have an **ESR** between 0 and 20 mm/hr.

Men under age 50 should have an **ESR** between 0 and 15 mm/hr.

Women over age 50 should have an **ESR** between 0 and 30 mm/hr.

Men over age 50 should have an **ESR** between 0 and 20 mm/hr.

Children should have an **ESR** between 0 and 10 mm/hr.

A common cause of ESR increase is: tissue Inflammation

Supplement Recommendations

The following supplements can help optimize and support the anti-inflammatory response in your system:

- Glutathione
- Turmeric/Curcumin
- Zinc
- Omega-3
- Huperzine

SPEAK WITH DR. STRONG

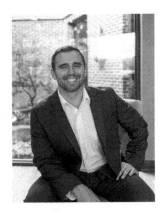

If you would like some help from me implementing strategies to help you with your health issues, then I'd like to invite you to speak with me personally.

You can work with me personally or look at my online health coaching course that gives you all the tools you need to thrive rather than merely survive.

Head over to: https://www.stronghealthplan.com/casestudy

There will be a short video and application about your health or what you need help with. (So we can review them before the call).

Answer the questions, and on the next page, you'll see a calendar with a list of available dates and times for your call. Pick the one that works best for you.

Once you have booked your time, the confirmation page will have some instructions on how to prepare for the call. Please review them thoroughly. Watch the video that breaks down what it looks like to work with me. Review the case studies from my clients. That way, when you get on the call, you will already have quite a few of your questions answered.

Once on the call, I will take a look at what you are doing, identify the problems you are having, and see if I can help. If I can help, I will show you what it looks like to work with me. You can then decide if you want to become one of my clients or not.

No pressure, but either way, you will get a lot of clarity out of this call. Visit https://www.stronghealthplan.com/casestudy to book your call today!

CONCLUSION

I hope this has been a valuable educational resource for you and has helped to demystify what all of the numbers and symbols on your bloodwork mean. If you haven't done a blood test yet, I encourage you to do so. Whether you've been struggling with chronic health conditions, or simply want to know where you stand – it's vital for understanding your baseline.

If you'd like more information and resources, I invite you to visit my site – www.stronghealthinstitute.com, and also engage with me on social media.

If you'd like to discuss your specific health goals and needs, you may also choose to schedule a consultation appointment on the site.

Take care!

- Dr. Todd Strong

Made in the USA
Middletown, DE
01 September 2022